Epilepsy in China: The AI Super Power

Authors and Contributors

Faisal Ahmed Shariff, M.Sc.

Mohammad Shueb, M.Sc.

Mohammed Aamir Niyaz, M.Sc.

Deepthi Shetty, M.Sc.

Copyright © Faisal Ahmed Shariff.

All rights reserved. No part of this publication may be reproduced, distributed, or transmitted in any form or by any means, including photocopying, recording, or other electronic or mechanical methods, without the prior written permission of the publisher, except in the case of brief quotations embodied in critical reviews and certain other non-commercial uses permitted by copyright law. For permission requests, write to the publisher, addressed "Attention: Permissions Coordinator," at the address below.

ISBN: 9798355285982

Imprint: Independently published

Any references to historical events, real people, or real places are used fictitiously. Names, characters, and places are products of the author's imagination.

Front cover image by Faisal Ahmed Shariff.

Book design by Faisal Ahmed Shariff.

First printing edition 2022.

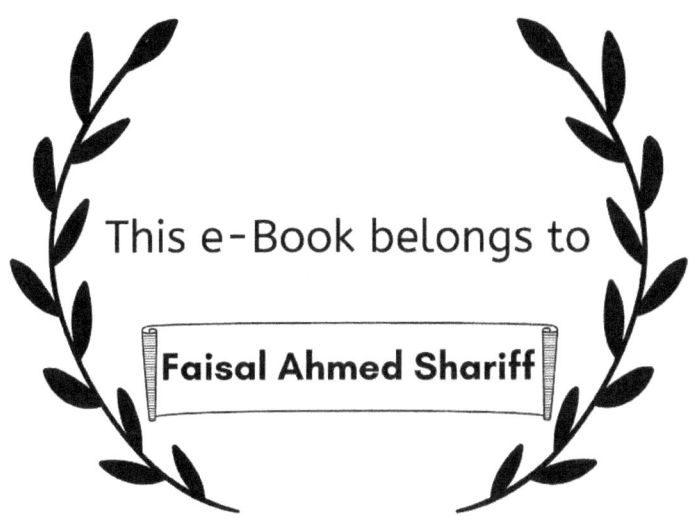

COPYRIGHT© 2022 BY FAISAL AHMED SHARIFF
ALL RIGHTS RESERVED

Contents

Epilepsy in China: The new approach 1
Authors and Contributors 1
CHAPTER 1: China the Super-power 7
   INTRODUCTION: 7
      TRADE: 11
      AGRICULTURE: 13
      The four great inventions of ancient China— 15
      Start-ups and Fundings 19
CHAPTER 2: AI and China, the two synonyms . 24
   AI in Drugs Discovery 40
CHAPTER 3: Is China Epilepsy ready? 45
   Survey Study 47
   Survey Study 48
   Survey Study 49
      Epilepsy awareness Campaign #1 50
      Epilepsy awareness Campaign #2 52
      Active Epilepsy: 53
      Untreated Epilepsy: 53
      Effective treatments: 53
      Treatment Gap: 54
      The following are the objectives of the extended National project: 56

CHAPTER 4: Drugs and Drug Manufacturers in China 57

    Vigabatrin: 61

    Brivaracetam: 62

    Fycompa: 64

- Sihuan Pharm: 66
- Changzhou Pharmaceutical Factory: 68
- HUAWEI: 69

    Pynegabine: 69

Pharma companies aiming to work on Epilepsy: 71

- Zhejiang Jiuzhou Pharmaceutical Co.,Ltd: 72
- NCPC INTERNATIONAL: 72
- Dingfukang Pharmaceutical Co.,Ltd: 73
- CSPC OUYI PHARMACEUTICAL CO., LTD: 73

CHAPTER 5: Orthodox Methods to treat epilepsy 75

Traditional Herbal Medicine 76

    Tai Chi 76

    Chinese Herbal Medicine 76

What does Science have to say with regards to TCM? 77

Chinese herbal Medicine in the treatment of epilepsy 78

Herbs used in CHM 83

Neuroscience in China 85

Chapter 6: Rise of the Chinese Healthcare system 89

Following points define the model of China's healthcare system 94

China's effort to control Chronic diseases have set a benchmark.. 96

Schemes and Programmes 98

Conclusion 100

CHAPTER 7: Anti-Epileptic drug discovery 102

Can AI help China outplay the world's top drug discovery researchers? 106

CADD 110

Current developments of Computer aided drug design... 115

Reference: 116

CHAPTER 1: China the Super-power

INTRODUCTION:

China, which is the largest country in Asia that spans an area of more than 3.7 million square miles. The majority of the nation is covered with mountains. The Trans-Himalaya, the Kunlun chain, and the Tien Shan are its three main ranges. Three major river systems can be found in China proper: "the Yangtze River (Chang Jiang), which is the third-longest river in the world at 2,432 mile (6,300 km), the Yellow River (Huang He), and the Pearl River (Zhu Jiang), which is 848 mile (2,197 km) long". It has a large Pacific Ocean coastline(Wu et al., 2004).

China has fourteen neighbours with whom it shares borders. Following is the list of countries which share borders: "Mongolia (4,630 km), Russia (4,133 km to the northeast and 46 km to the northwest), India (2,659 km), Myanmar (2,129 km), Kazakhstan (1,352 km), Nepal (1,389 km), North Korea (1,352 km), Vietnam (1,297 km), Kyrgyzstan (1,063 km), Tajikistan (477 km), Bhutan (477 km), Laos (475 km), Pakistan (438 km), and Afghanistan (438 km)".

One of the world's oldest cultures, China has made renowned contributions to a wide range of artistic, literary, architectural, and other fields. The Great Wall of China is the most well-known piece of Chinese architecture to listeners(Jin et al., 2004).

Chinese architecture is known for a variety of distinctive features; As many readers may be familiar with the use of notable structures. Particular stylings can differ significantly from regions across China. Chinese architecture has had a significant impact on nearby nations, and contact with the West only increased its global influence.

Like in the West, China's architecture has changed and evolved over time and in response to contact with other cultures. Early in the 20th century, Shanghai adopted many Western concepts to forge its own distinctive style, as evidenced by the renowned shikumen houses of the city. Additionally, the nation is home to many impressive examples of modern architecture, such as the National Stadium which is located in the capital of China, Beijing.

Not just the typical "Chinese food" you find throughout malls and shopping centres, but a whole treasure of cuisines with incredible depth and variety, China is well known for its culinary tradition. Anhui, Cantonese, Fujian, Hunan, Jiangsu, Shandong, Sichuan, and Zhejiang cuisines are the eight main types in China. There seem to be a lot more regional variation. Chinese cuisine has been infused with high significance and artistry all through history due to its diverse landscape, which ranges from tropical to desert to subarctic which in itself is quite a big deal. Chinese culture has long valued food as a vital component of a healthy lifestyle, and Chinese food therapy is still very well-liked today.

Chinese opera is respected and admired. There are more than 300 regional varieties of Chinese opera, with Peking (Beijing) opera being the most well-known, according to scholars Peter Lovrick and Wang-Ngai Siu. The most well-known types often feature elaborate costuming and staging. Even so, some aspects are less concerned with pageantry and might even be performed in casual attire. Jiang Qing, Mao Zedong's wife, promoted the Revolutionary Opera, a well-known example of this form. The term also covers what Westerners might refer to as ballet, such as the performance of Red Detachment of Women for Richard Nixon during his illustrious 1972 trip to China.

The nation has experienced consistent and brisk economic growth ever since Deng Xiaoping implemented new ideology and market reforms in the latter half of the 20th century. Depending on the metrics being used, China's economy is currently either the largest or second-largest in the world as of now. China ranks as the second-largest importer and exporter of goods in the world. China is expected to continue growing and is second only to the United States in terms of importance to the global economy. The middle class in China has grown significantly in recent years as the country moves further away from its past as an agricultural economy. China has also made huge progress in the creation and application of clean, renewable energy sources.

TRADE:

GDP/PPP: $14.72 trillion (2022 est.)

Growth Rate: 8.1% (2021 est.)

Inflation: 2.5% (2021 est.)

Government Revenues: 20.1% of GDP (2020 est.)

Public Debt: 45% of GDP (2020 est.)

Working Population: 774.71 million (2019 est.)

Note: by the end of 2012, China's working age population (15-64 years) was 1.004 billion

Employment by Occupation: Agriculture: 27.7%, Industry: 28.8%, Services: 43.5% (2016 est.)

Unemployment: 3.64% (2019 est.)

Population Below the Poverty Line: .6% (2019 est.)

Note: In 2011, China set a new poverty line at RMB 2300 (approximately US $400)

Total Exports: $2.732 trillion (2020 est.)

Major Exports which include electrical and other machinery, like computers and telecommunications equipment, apparel, furniture and textiles.

Export Partners: US 19%, Hong Kong 10%, Japan 6%, South Korea 4.5% (2017)

Total Imports: $2.362 trillion (2020 est.)

Major Imports that house electrical and other machinery, including integrated circuits and other computer components, oil and mineral fuels; optical and medical equipment, metal ores, motor vehicles.

Import Partners with their share in (%): South Korea 9%, Japan 8%, US 7%, Germany 7%, Australia 7%, Taiwan 6% (2019)

AGRICULTURE:

Major Industries such as Mining and mineral processing which includes iron, steel, aluminium, and other metals, coal; machine building; armaments; textiles and apparel; petroleum; cement; chemicals; fertiliser; consumer products (including footwear, toys, and electronics); food processing; transportation equipment, including aircraft, ships, and automobiles. Agricultural Goods: Rice, wheat, potatoes, corn, tobacco, peanuts, tea, apples, cotton, pork, mutton, eggs; fish, and shrimp (World leader in gross value of industrial output).

Resources: "Natural resources include uranium, aluminium, lead, zinc, rare earth elements, coal, iron ore, helium, petroleum, natural gas, ferrosilicon, bismuth, cobalt, cadmium, gallium, germanium, hafnium, indium, lithium, mercury, tantalum, tellurium, tin, titanium, tungsten, antimony, manganese, magnesium, molybdenum, selenium, strontium, vanadium"

Land Use: Forest: 22.3%, Other: 23%, Agricultural land: 54.7% (arable land 11.3%; permanent crops 1.6%; permanent pasture 41.8%); (2011 est.)

From the first century before Christ to the 15th century, China held the top spot in the world for the research of nature in many fields, with the four greatest inventions having the greatest global impact.

The four great inventions of ancient China—papermaking, printing, gunpowder, and the compass—were important contributions to global civilization.

The Paper:

The Paper was created in China for the first time. Before the invention of the paper the writings were carved on organic minerals such as grass stalks, earthen plates, tree leaves, sheepskins more astonishingly on bamboo, shells of tortoise and Ox shoulder blades. This was practices by Egyptians, Mesopotamians, Indians, Europeans and Chinese ancient people respectively. Following this, resident of ancient China was successful in producing the first type of silk paper also known as "Bo". after being inspired by the technique of silk reeling. But due to the lack of materials, it was very expensive to produce. A court official by the name of "Cai Lun" created a new form of paper with the help of bark, wheat stalks, rags and other similar materials in the first two centuries. It was more suited for brush writing, relatively inexpensive, light, thin, and sturdy.

Printing:

The Tang Dynasty printing the first book in history with a known printing date is a Buddhist sutra. Well before invention of printing, information was spread primarily through oral tradition or by handwritten manuscript copies. Both required effort and had few errors here and there. Stone-tablet rubbing became popular 2000 years ago during the Western Han Dynasty (206 B.C.–25 A.D.) it became common practise to engrave text or images on a wooden board, scribble it with ink, and then print them page by page on sheets of paper. Block printing came to be known as a result.

In the year 868, or nearly 600 years before that occurred in Europe, another amazing fact, that the first book published in China with a known date of Publication. Then this technology gradually made its way to China's neighbouring countries like Japan. Korea, Vietnam and Philippines which adapted the same. Later this technology migrated to Europe.

The Gun powder:

Ancient China is also credited with the invention of gunpowder. When ancient necromancers practised alchemy, they discovered that the right mixture of fuel and ores could cause an explosion when heated. This discovery led to the development of ash like substance later known to the world as gunpowder. Three recipes for gunpowder were documented in the Collection of the Most Important Military Techniques, "edited in 1044 by Zeng Gongliang". Gunpowder is an explosive mixture of saltpetre, sulphur, and charcoal. These have been identified by Dr. Needham as the original formulations of this kind. In the 12th and 14th centuries, respectively, the Arab world and Europe, the process of making powder was tried to introduce. The later development of gunpowder, originally used to make fireworks, revolutionised warfare all over the world.

The Compass:

Another significant invention from ancient China was the compass, a necessary navigational tool. People discovered a naturally occurring magnetite that attracted iron and pointed nowhere but north while mining ores and melting copper and iron. A round compass emerged after continuous improvement. "Dr. Needham cites Dream Pool Essays (1086)", written by Shen Kuo during the Song Dynasty, as one of the earliest books to discuss the magnetic compass. Alexander Neekam recorded the magnetic compass for the first time in

Europe in 1190. The introduction of the compass to Europe made it possible to navigate the world's oceans and sparked the discovery of the New World. "Francis Bacon", an English philosopher, wrote in his book "The New Instruments" that the invention of printing, gunpowder, and the compass had all changed the course of human history. He claimed that they had a greater influence on all of humanity than any empire, belief system, or celestial body(Xie et al., 2014).

Start-ups and Fundings

During the first half (H1) of 2022, 1,880 venture capital (VC) funding deals totalling $29.1 billion were disclosed in China. Nevertheless, this represents the highest capital raised by start-ups in any Asia-Pacific country during the period.

According to an analysis of GlobalData's Financial Deals Database, China's VC funding activity significantly increased month over month in June 2022. In contrast to the prior month, deal volume increased by 17.8% in June while the value of VC funding increased by 84%. The decline which was observed in some of the previous months, was not to affect by this growth, and as a result, there was YoY increase overall in H1 2022.

Chongqing Changan New Energy Vehicle: $785.7 million,

CanSemi: $671.43 million,

Innosecco: $472.5 million,

Jidu Auto: $400 million, and

Megarobo: Technologies $300 million in H1 2022 in China, among other notable VC funding deals.

Start-ups in China raised about $33 billion in the first eight months of 2020.

Although this sum is very similar to what it was during the same time period in 2019, fundraising was steady throughout the year. About $7.5 billion was raised by Chinese start-ups in the first three months. Although the funding increased to more than whopping $13.2B in the second quarter. Start-ups attracted nearly $12.2B in just July and August(Jinzhi & Carrick, 2019).

The start-up funding market experienced a lockdown in Q1, then recovered quickly, much like how China handled the COVID pandemic.

In 2020, a large portion of this funding went to start-ups offering distance learning/ E-learning and online medical care, both of which benefited greatly from the "new normal".(Men et al., 2019)

Chinese Start-ups which raised Billions of funds in Yuan (As of 2016)

- Didi Chuxing Technology – ¥477
- Ant Financial - ¥477
- Meituan Dianping - ¥349.8
- CATL – ¥147.4

- Lufax – ¥128.8

Chinese Start-ups which raised Billions of funds in Yuan (As of 2020)

- Qingju Danche – ¥106
- Yuanfudao – ¥106
- JD Health – ¥87.9
- Xingsheng Youxuan – ¥84.8
- Zouyebang – ¥79.5

There are 208 unicorn companies in China, most of which are concentrated in Beijing, Shanghai, Hangzhou, and Shenzen.

Top 10 Chinese Start-ups to watch out for;

- Geek+: Logistics and Robots for Warehouses - $439MM
- Full Truck Alliance/Huochebang: Uber Freight for China - $327MM

- Shannon AI: Fintech Focused AI - $16.8MM
- Hui'an Jinke (Ahi Fintech): Risk Management via AI - $15.3MM
- Video++: Video Streaming Services + AI Driven Advertising - $165MM
- Meiri Youxian/MissFresh: Instacart for China - $1.7B
- Starfield: Plant-Based Protein (Impossible Foods/Beyond Meat for China) - $10.1MM
- Chehaoduo: Car Trading Platform - $3.6B
- Yipin Shengxian/Yipin Fresh: Grocery Chain + WeChat-Based Delivery Series C: August 2020 ($382MM), Series B: March 2019 ($306MM), Series A: August 2018 (Not disclosed to public)
- Intellifusion: Visual Intelligence and AI - $184MM

CHAPTER 2: AI and China, the two synonyms

In China, where high tech, retail, and finance make up more than one-third of the country's AI market, AI adoption is currently high. For example, in the tech industry, market leaders "ByteDance" and "Alibaba", both well-known in China, are renowned for their online applications that are heavily dependent on artificial intelligence (AI).

Since China has the biggest online user base in the world and the ability to interact with consumers in various different ways to boost customer loyalty, revenue, and market valuations, the majority of AI applications that have been broadly accepted in

China till date have been used in consumer-facing industries.

According to researchers, China's new industries, including those in the automotive, transportation and logistics, manufacturing, enterprise software, healthcare, and life sciences, where innovation and R&D spending have historically lagged behind those in other countries, offer enormous opportunity for AI growth in the upcoming decade. There are many use cases in these industries where AI has the potential to generate up to $600 billion in economic value annually. ("To give an idea of scale, Shanghai, China's most populous city, had a GNP of roughly $680 billion in 2021, with a population of almost 28 million".) This value will originally come from sales of AI-based products.

The information and technologies that will support AI systems, the right talent and organisational mindsets to build such systems, new business models and partnerships to create data ecosystems, industry standards, and regulations are found in a huge number. Many of these, according to sources and international research done by various researchers, are becoming commonplace among businesses for extracting the greatest benefits from AI.

China's position as a leader in precise manufacturing for processors, chips, engines (All Insilico components), and other high-end components is changing its manufacturing reputation from one of being a low-cost manufacturing hub for toys and clothing. According to the research and available data, artificial intelligence (AI) can aid in facilitating this transition from manufacturing implementation to manufacturing innovation and generate $115 billion in economic worth.

The large percentage of this capital value ($100 billion) is probably going to be generated by the use of various AI technologies, like collaborative robotics, which will build the next-generation assembly line, which will replicate real-world assets for use in simulation.

Before starting large-scale production, manufacturers, suppliers of machinery and robotics, and companies that provide system automation are to simulate, test, and validate the results of manufacturing processes, such as product yield, in order to find expensive process early on which can also be seen as far-fetched goals. Wearable sensors are used been used by manufacturer to record hand and body movements in order to simulate human performance on the manufacturing line. After which, device setups and parameters are optimised.

Businesses with headquarters in China are undergoing digital and AI transformations. As a result, new local enterprise-software industries are emerging to support the required technological foundations.

Such companies' solutions are expected to generate an additional $80 billion. More than half of this value ($45 billion) is expected to come from cloud and AI tooling offerings.

For example, a local cloud provider provides over 100 local banks and insurance firms in China with an integrated data platform that enables them to work in both cloud and on-site environments while cutting the price of database design.

In a different scenario, a Chinese provider of AI tools has created a platform for an able to share AI algorithm that enables its data analysts to automatically train, forecast, and update the model for a specific prediction problem most prominently the weather. Hence the model production time was cut in half, from three months to about two weeks, thanks to the shared platform and integrated AI.

China has tremendously increased its investment in AI innovation in the healthcare and life sciences in recent times. By 2025, China's "14th Five-Year

Plan" is to increase R&D spending 7% annually, with at least 8% going toward basic research.

Accelerating drug discovery and improving success rates, which is a significant global issue, is one area of focus. Global pharmaceutical R&D spending increased by approximately 5% annually from $137 billion in 2012 to $212 -billion in 2021. The average time it takes to discover a new drug is 7.5 years, which not only prevents patients from getting the best therapeutic treatment but also reduces the length of the patent protection period. Only the top 20% of pharmaceutical companies around the world achieved a huge success on their R&D investments after seven years, despite higher success rates for developing new drugs.

Improving patient care is yet another top priority, and Chinese AI start-ups are currently working to establish their nation as one that provides healthcare that is more consistent and reliable in terms of diagnostic outcomes and clinical research.

The analysis indicates that faster drug discovery, clinical trial optimization, and clinical decision support are three specific areas where AI in R&D could add more than $25 billion in economic value. Further adding to this already plusher structure is Rapid drug discovery, Clinical trial optimization and clinical decision support.

How did China manage to outperform countries that had been working on this technology for much longer in order to build a world-leading AI research infrastructure in just two decades?

Data is required for the development of AI technology. Government data far outnumbers private sector data in numbers and scope in many aspects, and AI firms frequently gain access to such data when offering services to the nation(Allam et al., 2019).

Researchers say that such access can help advertising AI innovation in part because data and trained algorithms can be shared between government and commercial uses.(W. Qiu et al., 2018).

China measures the data available through contracts by measuring public intelligence services' capacity to collect surveillance video (CCTV), it is found that information contracts lead firms to develop noticeably and significantly more commercial AI software than data obtained from random sources without contracts(Hannas et al., 2022).

Not long ago, China was years, if not decades, behind the rest of the world. The United States leads the world in artificial intelligence. However, over the last three years, China has trapped the AI fever, going to experience a surge of enthusiasm for everything else we see in the world. AI energy has grown. Made its way over to government from the technology and business communities with a different approach as policy development.

This widespread support for the field had also shown and contributed to China's growing dominance in the field. Chinese AI firms and researchers have already gained significant hold on their American counterparts, playing with novel algorithms and business models that hold great promise to transform China's economy. These companies and academics have joined forces to elevate China to the status of true national AI superpower.

According to Ding, "China's plan to have globally leading AI companies by 2030 is also in reach, thanks to the growing expertise of its three core tech companies, Tencent, Baidu, and Alibaba". "These companies have become global leaders in AI," he says.

According to the New York-based research firm CB Insights, "China also has at least ten privately run

AI start-ups valued at more than US$ billion, including facial-recognition firm SenseTime".

According to Ma, "China's size of the population provides a large potential and unique opportunities to train AI systems, such as huge patient data sets for training software to predict disease".

AI differs from other technologies in several important ways. AI, unlike computer hardware or pharmaceutical / Drug development, is an open science. Many of the crucial algorithms in the field of AI have become public knowledge domains, accessible through published papers. Hence you can't potentially file a patent against that.

The most usual reason AI differs from traditional industries is in how profit is generated through innovation and improvised adaptations. Simply put, in AI research and data. Patents play an important role in securing firms' positions and protecting profit in traditional industries such as pharmaceuticals and mobile communications(J. Qiu, 2016).

Because AI is an open science as mentioned above, firms' competitive advantages are to those who has access to large set of data (Raw) and to develop specific knowledge or applications around the same interest (E.g.: Drug discovery) faster than anyone else.

China has a booming market that is open to new AI-based products, and Chinese companies are relatively quick to bring AI products and services onto the market. Chinese consumers are also quick to appreciate such products and services. As a result, they set an optimal environment for the rapid development of AI technologies and AI-powered products.

Quoting an example of the same "AI is frequently required to be improvised to specific business scenarios. You begin by creating a product (e.g., voice recognition or virtual speech texts). After which you attract a large number of users, who generate data. Finally, you use data to improve products using machine learning. This virtuous cycle results in advancements(X. Yang, 2019)".

Given the importance of large amounts of data to AI innovation, it's easy to see how China's massive market size explains its rapid AI catch-up. Because of the size of this industry, Chinese firms have potential to develop large databases.

When it comes to the medical field which has been particularly transformed, with a rise in health data by the availability of different modern-day technologies like Big Data, Machine Learning, Internet of Things (IoT), and Artificial Intelligence (AI). AI predictive tools are already being used in healthcare workforce recruitment and validation. One of them being speed of detection may it be any disease or any malfunction in the system(*AI Growth in China*, n.d.).

The speed of detection (here referred to as the process of disease identification) in the recent case of novel coronavirus (COVID-19), where its identity was done relatively earlier, All thanks to AI in China.

Human identification took only seven days, in contrast to previous outbreaks, such as the severe acute respiratory syndrome (SARS), which took four months.

However, it is worth noting that an AI-powered algorithm provided an early detection and warning on December 31, 2019, seven days before the World Health Organization (WHO) issued an official notice of the eruption SARS COV-2/COVID-19. Which again a big deal.

Talking of which, in a similar situation, an epidemic monitoring company called Metabiota was able to determine and alert that countries like Thailand, South Korea, Taiwan, and Japan were instantaneously susceptible to the coronavirus eruption just one week before it was officially confirmed in these nations using a predictive tool which again is with AI under the influence of China(*AI Leader China*, n.d.).

The adoption of AI-driven algorithms for early detection of pandemics is maturing and could be a powerful tool to better preparations in the near future. It is expected that as the accuracy of these instruments will improve and adapt over time with advancements.

As technologies advance, they will play a more crucial role in promoting the development of novel health policies.

Researches have shown how data and AI procedures aided in the early stages of the COVID-19 pandemic identification and offers initial supporting evidence to demonstrate that improved data sharing procedures will make a contribution to future urban healthcare policy, starting from China and expanding globally.

Countless authors agree on this belief and agree that processing of data using AI will greatly help new information that not only aid in the early diagnosis of pandemic outbreaks but will also be useful in protecting the country's economy from taking a hit when such pandemics occurs.

Not only China is well aware of the negative economic effects of SARS on their respective economies. All the nations across globe took a hit fighting the pandemic. As a result (Speaking of China), it appears that China's national level quick reaction to the novel coronavirus (COVID-19) through the suspension of internal China human movements, air flights, boats, and ferries, was successful.

Hence role of Artificial Intelligence (AI) in the early detection of the novel coronavirus (COVID-19) through the work of two companies, "BlueDot" (The company's system uses human and artificial intelligence to combine datasets with proprietary algorithms to deliver critical insights on the spread of infectious diseases, enabling governments, businesses, healthcare workers, and individuals to empower responses to infectious diseases) and "Metabiota"(Metabiota's team includes global leaders in epidemiology, veterinary medicine, laboratory science, data science, actuarial science, social science, and political economics, and serves some of the most respected customers in the corporate, insurance, government, and multilateral sectors) has shown how AI-driven algorithms can produce more accurate prediction and interpretations in the future through gradually increasing data.

On this basis, AI processes based on Smart sources of data science and their associated technological concepts, combined with wearables, can and should be encouraged, as they will result in larger datasets and thus more accurate prediction and identification overall(Roberts et al., 2021).

AI in Drugs Discovery

Artificial Intelligence (AI) playing a crucial role in the pharma companies is not particularly surprising. Chinese companies are using AI to produce more drugs(novel) and offer better services.

The nation is gaining rhythm for a boom in drug discovery supported by artificial intelligence. Industry experts and business leaders credit these companies' continuous improvement of their ecosystem to the nation's importance on innovation-driven development(*AI Drug Discovery*, n.d.).

China's dominance in AI-driven drug development is inevitable, despite the country's fairly late start (in the field). An end-to-end AI-driven drug discovery company, for instance, spoke publicly how AI has become central to its methodology and has a significant research and development team based in Shanghai, China. The administration of **ISM001-**

055, the first anti-fibrotic small molecule inhibitor produced by its AI-powered drug discovery platform for idiopathic pulmonary fibrosis, to a number of healthy volunteers in the phase-1 clinical trial to assess the safety (IPF). IPF should be noted as a progressive, chronic lung disease with unknown causes. It's a huge achievement because this is the first phase 1 clinical test of a drug created entirely with artificial intelligence.

Insilico (firm) used an AI platform to find the new anti-fibrotic target as well as the drug candidate. A drug target is a biological molecule, typically a protein, that is intrinsically linked to a specific disease and that a drug could target to have the preferred therapeutic effect. In a joint venture with a major Chinese pharmaceutical company, the company has also proposed a preclinical candidate compound for an innovative cancer immunotherapy(*AI and China*, n.d.).

According to a study from an industry dataset connected to a top online healthcare information provider, China almost doubled the amount of funding events and total financing value for AI-powered drug research and development in 2018. An enhanced working environment and rising market demand are the driving forces behind this. However, the report didn't disclose the precise numbers.

According to the report, 25 AI-powered drug discovery businesses in China received fresh funding in 2021. Another report claimed that China spent more than 8 billion yuan ($1.26 billion) last year on financing for AI-assisted drug discovery.

The use of AI in drug discovery has many benefits. Various R&D stages, including finding new drug targets and drug candidates, candidate optimization, and clinical research, are covered in detail by experts as to how AI technology could speed up new drug discovery and improvise the same. Even better, they continued, AI might lower research expenses and raise the likelihood that novel drugs will be discovered. China's infrastructure plays a significant part in these AI-driven businesses.

Over the past 20 years, the nation has built tremendous and jaw dropping infrastructures that can aid and test any new drug created anywhere to support drug discovery. Even better, the nation has noticeably lowered numerous regulatory barriers to carry out clinical trials, making businesses in China more willing to take chances for innovation and the development of new medicines.

As a result, AI-driven drug discovery firms are given new development innovations because it is expected that they will assist biotech and pharmaceutical firms in lowering the risks associated with new drug discovery. According to experts, only those biotechnological and pharmaceutical companies that use AI will succeed, despite how expensive developing new drugs is("Collaboration of Industry-Academia-Research-Application Improves the Healthy Development of Medical Imaging Artificial Intelligence Industry in China," 2019).

CHAPTER 3: Is China Epilepsy ready?

"Mini-ethnographic" studies which conducted in rural and urban parts of China to investigate the awareness and patients with epilepsy. Some emerging facts came into light with respect to computer-assisted data analysis. Epilepsy is a common and widespread neurological disorder, affecting people of all ages and socioeconomic classes all across the globe. There are approximately 9 million people with epilepsy in China, among them 6 million with active epilepsy(Campos, 2012).

The analysis tells of the current research on sources of stigma and factors of epilepsy. Data from 45 raw interviews and 8 focus group discussions which consisted of 6 people each were analysed to investigate people experienced epilepsy.(Bergin, 2011).

China which has the largest population of patients with epilepsy worldwide, hence the number of epilepsy centres has increased significantly in recent decades. Further which a nation-wide investigation on various aspects can bring in great value to the table which includes equipment, scale and distributions and epilepsy care capacity of each epilepsy care Center.(Y. Lin et al., 2021).

China which has approximately 10 million people affected by epilepsy. And which nearly has 20 different anti-seizure medications aiding that are the non-pharmacological options which are also available, keeping those aside there are still unmet needs (Beghi et al., 2019). (W. Z. Wang et al., 2003).

Following which a hierarchical model was then setup to include: Real life issues: approach towards the risk and costs of epilepsy; and ground Level issues. The analysis strengthens current research on factors and sources of the stigma of epilepsy(Thomas & Nair, 2011) and highlights issues for future practice.(R.-R. Yang et al., 2011).

Survey Study

The following study shows The World Health Organization (WHO) which collaborated with The Global Epilepsy Initiative launching an awareness campaign in collaboration with International League Against Epilepsy. This Awareness campaign in China against Epilepsy which included an epidemiological survey, an intervention trial and an educational programme. The main area of focus was Convulsive seizure treatment in Epileptic patients. The Primary care physicians appointed at the campaign prescribed phenobarbital (PB) (Drug), to almost half of the patients, by the end of the study which resulted in seizure free patients and no patient died because of any serious complications.

Survey Study

Epileptic patients of age 14 and permanent residents of rural Shanxi and Ningxia provinces were participants in this study, which was organised between May 2010 and June 2011.Few Trained local primary healthcare physicians made the first diagnosis by screening potential cases of convulsive epilepsy with an organised questionnaire. Potential positive screened individuals were then evaluated under the supervision of neurologist to confirm the on-going diagnosis.

Patients who met he following requirements were excluded from further studies which would have only increased problems rather come to a conclusion (e.g., seizures caused by drugs, alcohol, insomnia, febrile seizures, or pregnancy), people under the age of 14 at the time of this study which showed a progressive neurological condition, had co morbidities, hence other anti-epileptic drugs were as a result of polytherapy. Hence this same medical ethnic committee of China approved the study added all those took part have given their consents to Fudan University's Husashan Hospital which is located I Shanghai, China.

Survey Study

Epilepsy is a serious neurological disorder which has and is affecting people all across the globe. The distribution of which is spread equally throughout the world with more than 80% of it being affecting the people living in low- and middle-income countries. Further this study tries to estimate the burden of epilepsy in Mainland China from 1990 to 2015 and study how the burden travels by gender and age

Despite the significant advancements in economy and health services in China over the past few decades, the huge amount of information on the prevalence of epilepsy in Chinese bibliographic databases, while on the other hand with the help of Modelling approach/ Bioinformatic the burden is somewhat balanced. For example, using Meta-analysis method, which had the potential to discover 2.89% epilepsy prevalence in Mainland China.

For some reasons, researchers performed a systematic search of literature in both the databases i.e.; Chinese and English from 1990 to 2015, to examine the temporal variability and spatial variability of epilepsy prevalence in China which was also extended to how prevalence differed by gender and age.

Epilepsy awareness Campaign #1

The campaign was led by a door-to-door survey which was carried out in five provinces of China (Heilongjiang, Ningxia, Jiangsu, and Jiangxi).

Henan, Shanxi, and Jiangsu) in 2009, and then in Shanghai.

Random sampling/clusters were used studied in this survey which was based on Chinese census organised within province program areas.

A team of trained participating physicians and health workers from the Beijing Neurosurgical Institute who used a standard technique and screened 55616 people in total (I.e., 94.6% of the populations of the census units which were included in the study) following which they used a questionnaire with a specificity of 78.5% and a sheer sensitivity of 99.9%, the individuals who answered YES to any of the questions were examined by a neurologist at site to conform or to disprove the diagnosis.

Epilepsy awareness Campaign #2

Followed by which the second survey took place between September and December of 2004, post the therapies to see whether there was any effect to the treatment gap to observe any noticeable changes.

In the same survey, a census unit adjacent to that of the original unit was chosen each intervention area as mentioned above to prevent reporting bias. Following which in 2004, the total sample population was approximately 53796 with 51644 (i.e., 96%) of these people surveyed.

The technique and the methodology used in 2004 and 2000 survey respectively were the same. After the completion of the questionnaires, neurologists went onto visit each area and reviewed the medical history of each individual who had given a positive response to any of the questions in order to qualify for the final diagnosis. For ethical clearance The

Beijing Neurosurgical Institute's Institutional Ethics Committee reviewed the protocol and got the full clearance.

Below are the results of the survey which was keenly monitored and supervised by an inter-disciplinary team which studies all the aspects

Active Epilepsy:

Participants who have had two or more unprovoked seizures in the past 12 months following which they were considered to have active epilepsy

Untreated Epilepsy:

Untreated Epilepsy was defined as in any patient with active epilepsy who had not received any appropriate Anti-epileptic drug treatment in the week prior to the identification.

Effective treatments:

Effective treatments of active epilepsy which include treatment of underlying causes and diagnosis and well as the treatment for recurrent seizures using Anti-epileptic drug and surgery if necessary.

Treatment Gap:

This is represented by the percentage difference in the number of people with active epilepsy and the number of individuals whose seizures were being treated in a given population at a given point of time including human errors.(J. Sander, 2008).

Global Campaign Against Epilepsy which was ran from 2000 to 2004 which was to improve epilepsy care in rural China as a part of Demonstration Project.

This project included 5 provinces and a patient count of 2455 with phenobarbital monotherapy for convulsive epilepsy. In a year of span, roughly 40%

of the patients were seizure free, and then another 30% had their seizures reduced by more than half.

With the help of the Chinese Central government the campaign which started from 5 provinces has expanded to 12 provinces and 11,000 patients. Hence this is a step further for the implementation of a long-term goal to incorporate epilepsy management into China and its existing primary healthcare system. With the assistance of the Chinese central government, this initiative was expanded to 10 provinces in 2005.

The project which now involved 34 provinces with a collective population on 19 million people. More than 1500 country level doctors and village medical workers have been trained to manage the treatment to a whopping 459498 patients with convulsive epilepsy.

The project involved 34 provinces with a total population of 19 million people. More than 1,500 county-level doctors and village medical workers have been trained to manage the treatment of 459,498 patients with convulsive epilepsy.

The following are the objectives of the extended National project:

(1) to promote public and professional education on epilepsy.

(2) to improve diagnosis.

(3) To develop local campaigning and support groups for people with epilepsy.

(4) To decrease financial barriers to epilepsy services and treatment in rural areas and the social burden of epilepsy in rural areas.

(5) To develop and test a prototype for controlling general convulsive epileptic seizures using public health workers(W. Z. Wang et al., 2003).

CHAPTER 4: Drugs and Drug Manufacturers in China

The **Yangtze River Pharmaceutical Group** on October 15, 2021, (YRPG, founded in 1971, which is a national big-gun across regional pharma groups that has done some explicit research, industrial production and trading. China MIIT (Ministry of Industry and Information Technology), named its first innovative enterprises. YRPG, headquarters which is located in Taizhou (Jiangsu Province). Which has an employ strength of over 13000 people and is settled in an area spanning approximately 3 million square meters. Which also has more than 20 subsidiaries spread across China basically located in Beijing, Shanghai, Nanjing and Guangzhou. The revenue networks in linked throughout China.

For several years YRPG been working on its core basics which are its values of commitment and are dedicated to caring for all, adding that is supreme quality, great innovations, people oriented and sheer kindness. With this values YRPG has led Jiangsu pharmaceuticals industry in great profitable financial outcomes since 1996. While it is ranked fifth in the Chinese pharma industrial sector and is considered as one of the top 500 Chinese enterprises with one of the top 500 as tax payers

According to the data from MIIT (Ministry of Industry and Information Technology), YRPG ranked first in top 100 enterprises of the Chinese pharmaceuticals industries in three years i.e., 2010, 2014, 2015 and over that it was ranked first in the Chinese chemical pharmaceuticals industry four years consecutively and it was also named "2014 Chinese happy enterprise" and "2015 Quality benchmarking Enterprise". " In 2014 and 2015, YRPG was ranked as first in China Bio-Pharmaceutical plate for brand reputation, and further which brand value in China submitted the first marketing application for eslicarbazepine acetate which is also known as class 3 generic drug used for the treatment of Epilepsy.(Nishida et al., 2018).

Zebinix was approved in the Europe in 2009 which is considered as the first eslicarbazepine acetate originator. It is one of the epilepsy treatment choices that basically works by blocking the conduction of action potentials to inhibit or block the abnormal discharges released by the brain neurons respectively helping in controlling epileptic seizures. This drug has also been found to have shown good tolerance, high safety and a great efficacy after the administration for a prolonged time. But the native drug is yet to receive marketing clearance in China, nevertheless it was included in the market as second batch for recommended generic drugs, which was put up on the National Health Commission website on March 2021.

Eslicarbazepine Acetate which as above mentioned is an antiepileptic drug which is approved treatment for partial onset seizures as adjunctive therapy. Which is not thoroughly controlled with conventional therapy in United States, Europe and Canada. ESL which essentially is prodrug which is rapidly converted to active metabolites of eslicarbazepine. Thus, the action of mechanism is unknown and unclear but it is known to be having anticonvulsant activity inhibiting repeated neuronal firing and then stabilizing the inactivate state of voltage-gated sodium channels, which prevent the future activation of the seizures hence Yangtze River pharma group has backed this drug and is expected to be the first generic approved drug. Furthermore, a lot of other pharmaceuticals industries in China are trying to obtain the approval for the generic versions of ESL. Here is a point to consider where Eslicarbazepine acetate won't be the first generic drug used in counter for epilepsy to be out in the Chinese market as it will join forces with Vigabatrin, Brivaracetam and Fycompa.

Vigabatrin: Vigabatrin which has been recommended for the treatment of infantile spasms which basically occurs in children having sclerosis complex (TSC) as the first line aid, but there are other indications in children with TSC that are less well understood. As a survey ran where 201 children with tuberous sclerosis were screened and 21 children older than one year who were started on vigabatrin for any reason and showed adequate follow up data. Vigabatrin was prescribed for epileptic spasms to 13 individuals followed by tonic seizures to 5 individuals and status epilepticus for one. The average duration of treatment was 4 years. Hence as a result seizures were reduced to in all the individuals except one, where ten patients were seizure free the remaining four improved by more than 90%. Following which Vigabatrin was successfully given to 9 patients after 8 to 33 months after the first administration. The following changes were observed with rashes to 1 individual and behavioural decline to one, were reported as side effects(van der Poest Clement et al., 2018).

No retinal toxicity was reported in 14 patients with sufficient surveillance. Hence it was concluded that vigabatrin may be an effective therapy for the ones affected with epileptic spasms and tonic seizures.

Brivaracetam: This drug was approved by the US food and drug administration (FDA) dated February

19, and is primarily used to treat patients with partial seizures of age 16 years and above and also named as adjuvant treatment. As compared to the previously generation used drug which this drug now replaces with levetiracetam, the drug has similar chemical composition and action of mechanism, it is supposed to be the first AED which was approved by FDA for the treatment of partial seizures since 2013. Brivaracetam has a very high binding affinity and can specifically bind to synaptic vesicles protein 2A(SV2A), which is basically the activity site of AED levetiracetam. The efficacy of Brivaracetam is roughly 15-30 times that of Levetiracetam. Hence Brivaracetam is a new generation AED approved by FDA which is used for the treatment of partial seizures in epileptic patients of age 16 years and older, which can be used also in research lab and pharma development process.

Fycompa: Eisai Co., Ltd, which has recently announced their own in house discovered and developed AED known as Fycompa and the generic name known to the world is perampanel, hence fycompa has received two additional approvals in China as a Monotherapy for partial onset seizures and adjunctive treatments and as a monotherapy for paediatric indication for partial seizures where this drug is the combination of the previously mentioned Drugs (Above), as a result for the treatment for partial onset seizure with or without generalised seizures in patients with epilepsy with age 12 years and older, to bring this to notice that Fycompa has already received approval in China. With this approval, fycompa has open new ways for monotherapy and adjuvant therapy treatment for partial onset in China.(French et al., 2012).

Based on estimating monotherapy safety and efficacy in clinal studies of fycompa as an adjuvant therapy, following which various studies

304,305,306,355 were carried out throughout the world which included Europe, united States and China, this was carried out on patients age 12 and older with partial onset seizures, following this study the approval for monotherapy for partial onset seizures was granted, in addition to which the safety and efficacy information for Fycompa as monotherapy were the findings from a phase 3 clinical study. As epilepsy is thought to affect 9 million people in China and although it doesn't have a certain age group, as the attack of epilepsy is distributed to all the age groups.(Yamamoto et al., 2020).

At **Eisai's Tsukuba Research Laboratories** (The Tsukuba Research Laboratories which is a deep research centre for drug discovery research in the fields of neurology and oncology, the Tsukuba Research Laboratories will surely play an important role as a base for Data Driven Drug Discovery & Development (5D drug discovery).

Through the above-mentioned programmes and initiative, Eisai desires to speed up the process of drug discovery. And as also mentioned above the one daily tablet / monotherapy "Fycompa", was developed as the first in class- AED.

Some more core principles of Eisai are Neurology, which here is epilepsy, where Eisai will try to focus more on the area upfront. And they will try to prioritise the safety of the data and move in the notion of "Seizure freedom" to spread awareness epileptic patients all across the globe with the sheer success as Fycompa was approved as the monotherapy. Lastly the Pharma giants aim to address the various aspects and needs of epilepsy patients and their families to increase the awareness and meanwhile offer them benefits

However,

- **Sihuan Pharm:** Sihuan Pharmaceutical Holdings Group Ltd; The third business to obtain production approval for the Product in

China is Sihuan Pharmaceutical. The Product, which treats postherpetic neuralgia and epilepsy. Kids between the ages of 3 and 12 can use it as an adjuvant treatment for partial seizures.

- The oral administration of gabapentin capsules results in rapid absorption, good tolerance, very low toxicity and side effects which are so less that it can be neglected, and excellent therapeutic effect. It does not undergo metabolism, plasma protein binding, or liver enzyme induction when consumed. The drug can be used alone to treat generalised epilepsy or as a supplement to other anti-epileptic medications to treat refractory epilepsy because it can cross the BBB of the human brain with little chance of meddling with other anti-epileptic medications which might in worse case cause hindrance at a later stage. The Product is especially effective as a supplemented medication for epilepsy when compared to comparable products currently being used. Gabapentin capsules are now the first-line treatment for neuropathic pain due to their special benefits in this condition.

- **Changzhou Pharmaceutical Factory:** The Changzhou Pharmaceutical Factory (CPF), which is based in Changzhou, Jiangsu province, is one of China's top producers of pharmaceutical APIs and finished formulations. CPF was established in 1949. It has a 300,000m2 footprint and more than 1,450 employees, including more than 300 technicians with various specialties. With a focus on producing cardiovascular pharmaceuticals and medications, this company produces more than 3000 tonnes of 30 different types of APIs annually and more than 8,000 million tablets from 120 different types of finished formulations.

- HUAWEI: The term "Smart eye mask, device, health management method, and system" appears in a new health management patent published by Huawei on May 10 2021. The objective of Huawei's patent is to accurately diagnose, track, and report epilepsy disease.
- In accordance with the patent, data can be sent to a smart device connected to a Huawei smart eye mask when an epilepsy seizure is detected so that it can display the generated record. It should be noted that the smart eye mask has an EEG electrode, a signal acquisition unit, and a processing unit.

Pynegabine: The Shanghai Institute of Materia Medica (SIMM), Chinese Academy of Sciences (CAS), recently got approval from the State Food and Drug Administration (SFDA) for the clinical trial of **pynegabine tablet**, a first-class new anti-epileptic medication.

The FDA initially approved retigabine in 2011 as the first and only anti-epileptic medication. However, it is still under surveillance that some patients taking long-term medication might experience serious dose-related adverse effects, such as hyperpigmentation and the retina, primarily because of the medication's poor chemical stability and metabolic properties.

The research teams have been working on pyrenegabine as an anti-epileptic drug candidate for eight years, taking into account its pharmacodynamic safety and metabolic properties after several iterative structural optimization. Pyrenegabine has fully independent intellectual property rights because it targets the **potassium channel KCNQ**.

Pyrenegabine outperforms retigabine in terms of chemical stability and brain distribution, according to preclinical studies. Pyrenegabine also exhibits greater efficacy and positive results than that of retigabine in a number of animal models experiments, including a model for refractory epilepsy, in addition to lowering the risk of pigmentation.

Following additional clinical trials, it is hoped that pyrenegabine will emerge as a brand-new, Best/Only KCNQ modulator anti-epileptic medication. In the future, it might offer patients with refractory epilepsy new drug treatment options. All of these findings indicate that pyrenegabine will have promising development potential in future forth.

Pharma companies aiming to work on Epilepsy:

- **Zhejiang Jiuzhou Pharmaceutical Co.,Ltd:** A Chinese company called Zhejiang Jiuzhou Pharmaceutical Co.,Ltd. specialises in the novel development, production, and marketing of chemical Active Pharmaceutical Ingredients (API) and intermediate products. The Pharma Company primarily conducts business through two aspects: the Specialty APIs segment and Manufacturing Organization (CDMO) segment. The CDMO segment for new drugs and offers services for experimental drugs during pre-clinical trials.
- **NCPC INTERNATIONAL:** One of China's largest chemical and pharmaceutical firms, China Pharmaceutical Group is situated in the provincial capital of Hebei, Shijiazhuang. The North China Pharma Factory, which was established in June 1953 and began operating in June 1958, was the

forerunner of the major construction projects in China's "First Five" plan period. By making history by starting to produce antibiotics on a massive scale.

- Dingfukang Pharmaceutical Co.,Ltd: Dingkang Pharma, which was founded in the 1990s, has been granted permission by the China State Food and Drug Administration to sell chemical raw materials, amino acids, and pharmaceutical excipients. When building a better future for human health, Dingkang Pharma always strives for mutual development and upholds the principle of sustainable growth.

- **CSPC OUYI PHARMACEUTICAL CO., LTD:** A pharmaceutical company called CSPC Pharmaceutical Group Ltd (CSPC) sells novel, generic and bulk medications. The business develops, produces, and sells pharmaceuticals and related goods. The CSPC product line includes acarbose, penicillin sodium, cefazolin sodium, and meropenem, as well as capsules, tablets, injections, caffeine, and other antibiotics. In addition to ovarian cancer, breast cancer, high blood pressure, and childhood acute lymphoblastic leukaemia, the company also sells its products for other illnesses. Its medications concentrate on important therapeutic fields like neurology, diabetes, cardiovascular disease, oncology, and anti-infective. Asia, Europe, and the United States are where the company does business. The headquarters of CSPC Pharma are in Shijiazhuang, Hebei, China.

CHAPTER 5: Orthodox Methods to treat epilepsy

In recent times there has been a lot of buzz around numerous clinical studies and academic reviews which has shown the practise of traditional Chinese medicine including tai chi and herbal remedies. Tai chi being an example of psychological / a physical technique which has been used by the Chinese for a long time now, that was useful relief specific pain conditions and provide with a good quality of life. However, people have responded with mixed opinion on Chinese herbal medicines which even studies have proved and that applies to only a few such medicines not all.

Traditional Herbal Medicine

Tai Chi

In tai chi, specific positions, soft movements, mental concentration, breathing, as well as relaxation are combined.

According to research individuals who have got the treatment have shown great balance and stability mostly seen in elderly and patients with Parkinson's disease. This has also resulted in lessen knee osteoarthritis pain and with a significant effect (positively) on back pain.

Chinese Herbal Medicine

A survey which was conducted by NCCIH, found out one in every 5 Americans use Chinese herbal medicine, which have been used to treat various medical conditions including stroke, heart disease, mental disorders, Epilepsy and few respiratory diseases namely bronchitis, common cold. Yet no definite conclusions about the efficacy of many studies can be drawn because of their low quality.

What does Science have to say with regards to TCM?

There are numerous safety concerns with the herbal medicine used in TCM, according to reports and studies. The list is as follows:

Unwanted or unnecessary animal or plant source materials, which include Drugs, heavy metals, pesticides (Sulphites), which could potentially cause asthma or some adverse allergic reactions without proper use herbal medicines or may be using incorrect herbs to treat disease which is not even related to it may cause some serious issues like organ damage and this has been found in some present day Chinese herbal medicines.(C.-H. Lin & Hsieh, 2021).

The above-mentioned study was funded by NCCIH.

Chinese herbal Medicine in the treatment of epilepsy

For over thousands of years CHM has been in use for the treatment of Epilepsy and seizures. The foundation of TCM is the idea that food and medicine have the same origin, then why not people include herbal medicine in the daily diet just like the idea of Ayurveda in India which resembles the same principle. This is also referred to as the medical diet therapy, as it is included in the natural diet. The idea behind this diet therapy is to use food as a form of therapy for illness.

Recent studies have also shown that CHMs are effective. CHM is individualised medicine that is prescribed based on the Chinese medical system's constitution theory to promote health and treat illnesses. As a result, different herbal treatments for the same diagnosis may be given to different people.

Dietary therapy used in traditional Chinese medicine seems to be both secure and efficient Looking through article published on PubMed dated November 2020, which refer the use of conventional Chinese Medicine which includes plants, fungi and animals in clinical settings. Through a variety of methods and mechanism like antioxidation, GABAergic effect, anti-inflammatory effect, modulation and regulation of NMDA channels, potassium channels and sodium channels and lastly neuroprotection, combination of different herbs can result in the increase of antiepileptic effect

In most of the cases medication is the primary method of treatment for epilepsy, but other treatments like functional surgery have its own sweet share. To control the electric firing of the neurons, the present time approved anti-epileptic medications are mainly targeting voltage-gated ion channels like sodium, calcium and potassium channels.

Carbamazepine, Phenytoin, valproate, retigabine, ethosuximide and zonisamide are currently being used. Going in a bit of detail, to increase the synaptic inhibition, some medications which include carbamazepine, benzodiazepines and tiagabine are used which act on the GABA transporters and GABA receptors. Vigabatrin inhibits the GABA transaminase which as a result lowers the GABA metabolism, in order to reduce synaptic excitation, some medications inhibit NMDA receptors such as Perampanel (Fycompa in

China) and topiramate, which acts on the AMPA glutamate or kainite receptors.

There are many herbal remedies that have shown anti-epileptic properties. Such as Ginkgo biloba and Huperzia Serrata. While Cannabidiol is the first anti-epileptic drug which was derived from a plant, and was approved by the FDA (USA) in the year 2018 to treat Lennox-Gastaunt syndrome and Dravet syndrome. Cannabidiol has proven to be effective and safe under the extensive research. But the fact that the technique underlying the anti-epileptic effect is not fully understood, despite this numerous clinical trials have demonstrated its potential for use in medicine.(Minamil et al., 1999).

Anti-epileptic medications can depict a negative impact on a patient's quality of life in terms of side effects. In a recent review article, four problems with anti-epileptic medications were categorised as follows: general side effects, psychological problems, social problems, and economic problems. Severe psychiatric, cognitive, behavioural, endocrine, and dermatological diseases and dysfunctions are examples of antiepileptic drug side effects. The medications may have an impact on how well patients perform academically, vocationally, at work, and interpersonally. Increasing the dosage of anti-epileptic medications is associated with depression and suicidal thoughts. Some people who need long-term treatment for epilepsy stop taking the expensive and difficult-to-get anti-epileptic medications. Especially in developing nations, these difficulties cause patients to refuse Western medical care. Otherwise, despite the fact that numerous novel anti-epilepsy medications have been created in the past 20 years, about one-third of patients lack adequate seizure control because of they lacked awareness as to how COVID-19 was to people during the initial phase.(Q. Li et al., 2014).

Nature/Natural source medicines have been found to be more effective at treating epilepsy with fewer side effects. The regulation and modulation of synapses, receptors, and ion channels, the prevention the of inflammatory effect, and the control of the immune system are just a few of the reported mechanisms of natural medicine. Patients have subconscious fear of the adverse effects of Western medicine / surgery is what has caused a trend toward turning to traditional Chinese medicine for treatment. Traditional herbal medicine may also be more affordable and available to patients than conventional therapies(J. W. Sander & Shorvon, 1996).

Herbs used in CHM

- Gastrodia elata
- Uncaria rhynchophylla
- Acori tatarinowii

- Paeonia lactiflora
- Bupleurum chinense
- Ziziphus jujuba
- Pinellia ternate
- Paeonia suffruticosa
- Stephania tetrandra
- Cistanche deserticola
- Corydalis yanhusuo
- Salvia miltiorrhiza
- Ganoderma lucidum
- Buthus martensii

Anti-epileptic drug and herbal combined effect therapies are becoming more and more popular and acceptable today. With the hike in complications, components in a number of herbs used in a Chinese medicine formula, it can be challenging to confirm an herb-drug interaction. Some natural herbs have been reported to enhance the anti-convulsant effects of anti-epileptic medications. Few studies have examined the potential interactions between herbs and drugs(C.-H. Lin & Hsieh, 2021).

According to those studies, natural remedies, the majority of which are basically derivatives plants and herbs, can increase the effectiveness of anti-epileptic medications. Few studies mentioned in this review article, Chinese medicine demonstrated a beneficial effect when used in combination with Western medicine.

Chinese medicine is comprehensive and can be tailored to each patient's symptoms. With the use of TCM in medical diet therapy has become widespread. Some nations, particularly in the East, use herbal medicine as either a primary or complementary form of treatment. The use of herbal medicine will likely move in the direction of evidence-based practise(Q. Wang, 1996).

Neuroscience in China

After quite some time, nearly two decades of economic boom, China has been more focused on science like never before, aiding which is Neuroscience that has dedicated immensely in this field. The establishment of Chinese society for Neuroscience which was in the year 1995, where the rapid expansion phase was at its fullest of pace, science funding in China has increased quite significantly in the first decade of the century with an increase of 20% speaking of 2011, thus the ION (Institute of Neuroscience) founded in 1999 arrived at the sweetest of times to serve as the key role in the rapidly growing research community.

This is made successful only because many young researchers and scientist who were trained in the US and Europe made their way back to China their native country and one of them being Fang who got a PhD in the year 2007 from the university of Minnesota, and serves the purpose of a group's leader at the Perking or Beijing university using various imaging methods.

Beijing university which is located in the capital of China, is one of the renowned universities of the nation, which houses 12000 undergraduates and master's students, and over 7000 PhD students. He mainly receives the research fundings from the two supremely major funding organisations i.e., "National science Foundation of China" (NSFC) and "the ministry of Science and Technology" (MOST).

In the process of advancement, one such study was enough to make China outshine others i.e., Pain research and Brain, as they have studied the molecular analysis of long-term pain. Researchers have also gained a lot more detailed picture of the "molecular mechanisms of the transmission of pain". Zhang's group which was keenly working on this mechanism has found leads and discovered a new regulatory cum modulatory system which involves the protein Follistatin-like-1 (FSTL1), which is supposedly the first "endogenous activator" of a sodium pump that was discovered within the human body, which helps in the regulation of the synaptic transmission.

Moreover, that this is considered as an important neuromodulator and novel neurotransmission mechanism which is first in China. Following this success, the researchers in China are now on the move to find the transmission of pain in the brain and the pathways which are related to it. One more point to consider, while the processing of pain at the periphery and spinal cord is well studies by the researchers, its impact/effect in the brain are yet to be explored.

To sum it up Chinese and foreign researchers have been finding ways to approach it in a different way. This is surely a positive sign for neuroscience as much other fields which go hand in hand.

One more area of interest is the ion channels which could potentially be the reason for rapid changes in membrane potential of synaptic transmission and which will surely be essential for a variety of neuronal functions. The researchers have contributed heavily to discovery the importance of ion channels in neuronal survivals.

Chapter 6: Rise of the Chinese Healthcare system

China which is rapidly developing country which has a massive population of 1.45 billion people. Hence Chinese government was always keen in improving the already best in class healthcare and medical services, to help transform the development model of the Chinese health sector one step ahead its league.

China which had roughly 3650 medical and health institutions, just about 541000 healthcare staff and a bed capacity of 85000 at health institutions, following which the average life expectancy in China was a mere 35 years. To counter this situation, the government put in great effort to transform the medical and healthcare sector and by revamping its services. They also implemented guidelines which had no stigma and hence the idea was to serve a large portion of the population. Incorporating these changes had quite a significant positive impact, that greatly enhanced people's health and major achievements were made by the medical sciences post applying the changes.

Following this Chinese scientists were the first to identify Chlamydia trachomatis, couple of more achievements that Chinese portraited in this field were "world's first severed limb replantation and Artemisinin which is an effective cure for malaria was first identified in the Chinese laboratory.

China again revamped the medical and healthcare system in 2009 to adapt the new needs and changes. Which this changes one such strong and more stressed statement was that basic medical and healthcare system/ facilities should be available to all the citizens in the form of public product. This portraited the non-profit nature of the Chinese government and they were serious about the reform.

The listeners should know that China has proposed the implementation of the Four systems and they are, "Public health", "Medical services", "Medical Security" and "Drug supply", and supporting that they launched Eight supporting mechanisms such as "Medical and healthcare management", "operation", "investment", "pricing", "supervision", " technology and personnel management" and " law based management", was an effort put up by the Chinese government to evenly spread the basic medical and healthcare system and to prosper the overall development of the sector.

More improvements were made in the Medical and healthcare system during 2009-11, Thus during the next five-year plan i.e., 12th (2011-15), the government adapted ways to accelerate the basic medical system and improve community-level healthcare services and made sure the equal access to basic public medical and health services were availed.

Just after a year of implementation, China had doubled the effort to bring a renovation in the medical and healthcare system. China has also implemented some serious illness insurance policies which included residents from both Urban and Rural areas. Aiding that was the enhanced multi-layer diagnosis and treatment system.

China issued "Healthy China 2030" on 30th October 2016, the initiative behind the cause was to promote public health and fitness awareness, with plans to make the Chinese healthier.

All the policies and improvisation provided Chinese healthcare system with a huge success, where the average life expectancy rose to 76.5 year (2016) from a mere 35 years in (1990). Mortality rate dropped from 88.9/100000 persons (1990) to 19.9/100000 persons (2016). These reforms have definitely shaped the Medical and Healthcare services/system in a very productive way within a short span of time, China was able to achieve World's largest network of basic medical insurance which covers all the citizens of China, patients with serious illness/ Diseases were provided with insurance, availability of emergency medical services and aiding that was an improved medical assistance.

In 2015, China set up a world record by creating the world's Largest online direct reporting system for public health emergencies and notifying epidemics. During the initial runs the average reporting time was 5 days which was reduced to 4 hours while it was introduced to public.

With this significant progress the development of Medical and Healthcare system has reached new hights with over 980000 medical and health institutions at various levels, 11 million health working personals and about 7 million beds at hospitals. After sheer hard work and immense effort, China's medical and health services have reached new hights.

Following points define the model of China's healthcare system

- Focusing on Health and Fitness – China's government has always prioritized people's health and is keenly working on its development strategies; they have come up with exclusive health and fitness policies in motivating the individuals.

- Prevention is better than cure – To move from orthodox way of treatment i.e., migrate from treating illness to boost people's health. The focus is also out on prevention of diseases and its treatment accordingly and synchronised working for both brain and body. Western medicine and TCM are made to work parallelly. Some serious efforts have been made to prevent and control chronic and endemic diseases. To get more insights of occurrence of illness, the medical sector is studying the patterns related to health issues, focus on early diagnosis.

- Non-profit Services – The idea is to make all the basic medical and healthcare services available for all the citizens. As public hospitals play a vital role in the development of public healthcare sector, steps have been taken to ensure the end-to-end access to these hospitals.

- Equality to all – China is focused on providing medical and healthcare services coverage throughout the nation, primarily focusing on rural areas and native communities, to cover the gaps between urban and rural healthcare sectors which makes everything linear.

China's effort to control Chronic diseases have set a benchmark

Monitoring network has been setup in China to control chronic diseases and reduce the risk factor. As mentioned, numerous times in this book, the basic public health services are provided free to elderly patients with hypertension or diabetes. There are various services like screening of cardiovascular diseases, oral disease screening and most prominent being the early diagnosis and treatment of Cancer.

A statistic shows, by the end of 2016, the screening services for cardiovascular diseases has been done to over 6.1 million people, for which 820000 were prone to high risk and 952000 follow ups were organised.

Around 2.14 million people who were at high risk of cancer were given early diagnosis and treatment. Nearly 55000 patients were diagnosed, and the diagnosis rate reached a whopping 80%.

Schemes and Programmes

China is dedicated to raise the standard and effectiveness of medical services, while also making it easily accessible. It strives to strengthen the medicine supply chain and focus on the development of well-integrated medical and healthcare services system.

The health care system in China is made up of various schemes, that work together to serve the entire population. Employees in the public sector are provided with free medical services, a non-contributory programme which started way back in 1952 to pay 100% of the medical expenses. Those employees reside in the Urban areas are aided with Basic medical insurance which provides coverage under the "Urban Employee Basic Medical Insurance" (UEBMI).

UEBMI is a contributory programme that pays around 64% of claimants' medical expenses. In turn it requires 6% contribution from employers and 2% from employees. Urban residents without jobs are eligible for coverage through the Urban Residence Basic Medical Insurance (URBMI) programme as said earlier, which covers about 50% of the medical costs in exchange for small contributions.

Furthermore, the Medical Assistance for Urban Residents (MAUR) scheme, a non-contributory programme established in 2005 to offer subsidies for members to pay into MIUR or receive direct assistance, allows low-income urban residents access to health care. China's rural people are covered by several programmes, such as the New Co-operative Medical Scheme (NCMS), which was initiated in 2003 and pays for roughly 50% of the claimant's medical expenses. The Medical Assistance for Rural Residents scheme, which is designed similarly to the MAUR programme and offers rural residents a subsidy to join the NCMS or receive direct assistance, is a complementary programme to this one.

Conclusion

The Chinese government genuinely respects and values the right of the people to good health, and it sees maintaining that right as a fundamental duty of government. Important steps have been taken with the intention of helping people now and in the future. China has made a significant contribution to humankind's sustainable development in the field of health care.

As China has come up with certain schemes to safeguard people's right to health initiative. They have a long-term goal of building a healthy China. Aiding is a series of plans, Schemes and policies such as "Healthy China 2030", the national fitness program (2016-20), the 13th year five-year plan for medical and health services development.

The Chinese government has come up with a trajectory, showing their "Goals" set for future, one of which being able to efficient and effective treatment, which spreads across the nation from Urban to rural areas and providing the residents of both the sectors with right to health, which they have achieved in 2020 during the high time of COVID-19. The plan for 2030 is to enhance the health-promotion system, and tally it with other developed countries Government is dedicated to comprehensively safeguard people's health and promote overall development of healthcare system with at most priority.

CHAPTER 7: Anti-Epileptic drug discovery

Phenobarbital which was invented in 1912 was the beginning of the epilepsy treatment in the modern era. Another thing worth noting is the significant development was the invention of phenytoin which was introduced in the late 1930s, which came courtesy to the animal models developed for the tracking of antiseizure activity. The same idea/designs were important in the later development of numerous other anti-seizure drugs (ASMs). Today, there are more than 30 medications against epilepsy.

These medications had a lot of things to offer, one of which being the improvised customisation treatment which was designed different for each individual's needs because of the variation in pharmacokinetics, toxicity, efficacy and side effects.

Some of the ASMs that were developed after 1985, or better called as the second-generation of ASMs, had some safety advantages over older generation medications, and hence they haven't significantly increased the percentage of patients who are completely seizure-free.

There are significantly less specialists and neurological sectors and facilities as compared to other big nations which treats a large number of populations affected by active epilepsy nevertheless the Chinese government is working in the right direction to spread awareness.

China conducted The Global campaign against Epilepsy Demonstration project, which was sponsored by WHO in 2002.

The Global Campaign against Epilepsy (GCAE) Demonstration Project, sponsored by WHO in 2002 and conducted in China, evaluated the core for providing appropriate epilepsy management in primary care settings. As the Chinese government went on to fully support the campaign and The Chinese government expanded the initiative to more locations across the country as a result of the project's success.

A noticeable Spike in economic expansion over the past 20 years, there has been a rush in a positive way for the development of clinical treatment and research for epilepsy in China. There was a comparative treatment gap in "traditional" areas of China where epilepsy was not recognised as a medical condition but the issue has been in keen observation since the hike in epileptic patients. Epilepsy treatment is continuously advancing in "modern" China, where top notch clinical and surgical care is provided alongside advance scientific research.

In 2005, the International League against Epilepsy (ILAE) and the International Bureau for Epilepsy (IBE) accepted the China Association against Epilepsy (CAAE) (www.caae.org.cn)

By 2018, there were around 28 branches of CAAE, and their active members had surpassed 10,000. CAAE has played a significant role in igniting epilepsy interest in China over the past ten years. There has been a strong push to advance professional care, and there have been campaigns to lessen misconceptions, stigma, and discrimination surrounding epilepsy, which may have helped to close the treatment gap and is considered as a masterstroke played by the Chinese government. Centres in China have conducted research in this area, and some ground-breaking results have also been published(L. Wang, 2018).

The most prominent form/type of drug resistant epilepsy is studied to be the temporal lobe epilepsy (TLE), with hippocampal sclerosis. Recent Chinese research examined potential TLE mechanisms, particularly the role of microRNA in regulation (miRNA). In order to better understand the origin of epilepsy and develop more effective treatments,

Chinese researchers have been working hard to create new and enhanced animal models of epilepsy.

In China over the past decade, significant progress has been made in the study of seizure disorders.

And in the year 2018, China had just over 5000 reports published in English and an equal number journals published in Chinese. With funding primarily provided by the National Natural Science Foundation, the Key Research Study Program of the Ministry of Science and Technology, and the National Health Commission, China is currently one of the top ten nations in the world for epilepsy research output(J. Yang, 2013).

Can AI help China outplay the world's top drug discovery researchers?

The drug discovery in China has started somewhat slowly compared to many other nations, but the size of the Chinese pharmaceutical market is among the top three globally. In China, more thorough drug discovery research is at surge (Currently). With the help of AI, a machine can perform tasks as well as or better than a human. With numerous new AI-powered drug discovery businesses emerging in China

Drug discovery involves a series of processes that, in general, fall into two categories: preclinical and clinical stages. Preclinical trials, hit discovery, and validation of targets are all included in the preclinical phase.

The crucial document known as the IND (Investigational New Drug) defines the line between the preclinical and clinical stages. The approval of an IND application is a significant step in the drug discovery process because it advances the investigation into the clinical phase, where trials and experiments are carried out on real subjects.

According to available data, a new drug on an average takes about 10 years to develop from its initial discovery to the final product launch. And the estimated price is generally at least USD 1 billion. Less than 10% of the numerous drug research projects reach the clinical trial stage. Additionally, more than half of the candidates will be eliminated during the clinical trial screening. Only a small proportion of candidates will be turned into a product and sold.

The incidence of diseases like cancer, diabetes, and other chronic illnesses as well as Epilepsy is rising each year in China as a result of the country's rapidly ageing population, altered dietary practises, and work demands as in most other countries. The percentage of people in China who are 65 or older and older than 14%, according to the most recent national census, shows that China has officially embraced an ageing society. To address these unmet medical needs, there has been an increasing need for novel medications and cutting-edge pharmaceutical R&D.

By 2023, the pharmaceutical market in China is predicted to grow to USD 161.8 billion and account for 30% of the global market, second only to the United States. However, the majority of medications on the market right now are either generic versions or were created outside of China.(Y. Li et al., 2021).

The Chinese cabinet, the State Council, overhauled the system for reviewing and approving medications in 2015 by clearing the backlog of older applications, particularly for redundant generics. Additionally, it established a special procedure for the review and evaluation of novel drugs with urgent clinical requirements, which promoted and sped up the development of novel drugs in China. Which has caught a rapid pace after the most difficult barrier was removed, China-based novel drug companies began to emerge and attract investors' attention(Ahmed et al., 2021).

CADD

Computer-aided drug design (CADD) is essential to the discovery and improvement of lead compounds when developing new drugs. Advancements of Traditional Chinese Medicine (TCM) is a successful strategy for finding new drug targets and developing new medications (PDTs). The "bottleneck" that has obstructed the development of new drugs in the discovery, profiling and validation of post deposition treatments PTDs, which has been addressed and resolved. Innovative drug research has a lot of potential and is very important(Y. Li et al., 2021).

"Druggability" and "specificity" of PTDs, the "druglikeness" of drug candidates, were the two most important aspects of discovery and validation. Realizing the "from gene to drug" invention and innovation strategy is crucial. By combining alternative high-new technology, particularly CADD, researchers have been able to find the perfect sweet spot and find innovative solutions that are in line with the development of the nation.

The struggle against disease also has a long history in human history. More and more incurable diseases are now on the verge of being cured cheers to the quick reaction and development of life science and biotechnologies like gene editing NGS and deep sequencing.

Therefore, it is crucial to establish the synergy between various driving forces when developing new drugs. China, the most populous nation on earth, has the highest prevalence of a wide range of novel diseases, creating a special environment for biomedical research and the development of new disease therapies which the whole world can adapt.

Although the majority of Chinese pharmaceutical firms have historically concentrated on producing generic medications, some efforts to develop first-in-class medications are beginning to initiate, particularly for small-molecule medications.

There are several methods for creating new medications. First being the high-throughput screening (HTPs) which is a key method for discovering first class drugs that does not strictly require knowing the structure of the drug targets. Large pharmaceutical companies are using their own libraries (compiled with their own data) which frequently contain millions of tiny molecules also can be considered as potential lead or hit molecule for high-throughput screening.

CADD (computer Aided Drug Discovery or Computer Driven Drug Discovery) could significantly accelerate the drug discovery process while lowering the cost of R&D. The modern use of molecular dynamic simulations (MDS) and other

CADD technique used in the process of drug discover which according to Drug Discovery World, shortens the R&D cycle by about 0.9 years and saves about 0.15 billion dollars for each new drug developed which is quite a big deal, demonstrating that drug design has evolved into a crucial part of drug innovation which in itself is a huge number. It is not wrong to say that "computing" is in-built throughout the process of developing pharmaceuticals, from the get go like target identification to lead compound discovery/ identification and further optimization to preclinical toxicology and dynamics studies of pharmaceuticals, preclinical drug efficacy tests, and even clinical trials.(Ahmed et al., 2021)

The first successful drug of multiple targets created with the aid of CADD is the "integrase inhibitors" for the treatment of HIV. Over 10,000 possible targets in a cell have been identified as potential drug targets, and CADD would be an effective way to screen potential drug candidates, further optimise their structure, and confirm their activity. CADD was used in the design of more than 50 drugs, and there are still more in clinical trials.

A class of medications known as biologics (or biopharmaceuticals) is based on proteins and has therapeutic effects. CADD is very much skilled at creating antibody-drug conjugates (ADCs), that combines an antibody with a biologically cytotoxic small molecule for the purpose of treating cancer. Hence a signal is released by the antibody of ADCs to a specific tumour marker, which causes the tumour cell to absorb the ADCs. The cytotoxic substance would dissolve/kill the cancerous cell in this manner. It is crucial to attach the molecule to the antibody at the proper location without affecting the ADCs' ability to be recognised and absorbed. It is a hefty task in drug development. Particularly in the areas of epitope recognition and antibody design, CADD has significantly made progress in assisting protein drug design. To carry out the task, there are actually good software available both freeware and commercial tools(L. Wang, 2018).

Current developments of Computer aided drug design

1. Structure based drug design
2. Protein structure determination
    2.1. Homology modelling
    2.2. Folding recognition
    2.3. Ab initio protein modelling
    2.4. Hot spot prediction
3. Docking
    3.1. Autodock
    3.2. CDOCKER
    3.3. Flexible docking
    3.4. Transmembrane protein modelling
    3.5. Binding free energy
    3.6. Flexibility of protein ligand complex

   3.7. De novo evolution
4. Ligand-based drug design
5. Quantitative structure - activity relationship (QSAR)
      5.1. CoMFA
      5.2. CoMSIA
6. Molecular Dynamics Simulations
7. Lead optimization

Reference:

Ahmed, H., Khan, M. A., Ali Zaidi, S. A., & Muhammad, S. (2021). In Silico and In Vivo: Evaluating the Therapeutic Potential of Kaempferol, Quercetin, and Catechin to Treat Chronic Epilepsy in a Rat Model. *Frontiers in Bioengineering and Biotechnology*, *9*. https://doi.org/10.3389/fbioe.2021.754952

AI and China. (n.d.). https://www.chinadaily.com.cn/a/202206/23/WS62b3c9eea310fd2b29e680dc.html

AI drug discovery. (n.d.). https://equalocean.com/analysis/2022070818467

AI growth in China. (n.d.). https://www.theverge.com/2021/3/3/22310840/ai-research-global-growth-china-us-paper-citations-index-report-2020

AI leader China. (n.d.). https://www.nature.com/articles/d41586-019-02360-7

Allam, Z., Tegally, H., & Thondoo, M. (2019). Redefining the Use of Big Data in Urban Health for Increased Liveability in Smart Cities. *Smart Cities*, *2*(2), 259–268. https://doi.org/10.3390/smartcities2020017

Beghi, E., Giussani, G., Nichols, E., Abd-Allah, F., Abdela, J., Abdelalim, A., Abraha, H. N., Adib, M.

G., Agrawal, S., Alahdab, F., Awasthi, A., Ayele, Y., Barboza, M. A., Belachew, A. B., Biadgo, B., Bijani, A., Bitew, H., Carvalho, F., Chaiah, Y., ... Murray, C. J. L. (2019). Global, regional, and national burden of epilepsy, 1990–2016: a systematic analysis for the Global Burden of Disease Study 2016. *The Lancet Neurology, 18*(4), 357–375. https://doi.org/10.1016/S1474-4422(18)30454-X

Bergin, M. (2011). NVivo 8 and consistency in data analysis: reflecting on the use of a qualitative data analysis program. *Nurse Researcher, 18*(3), 6–12. https://doi.org/10.7748/nr2011.04.18.3.6.c8457

Campos, M. G. (2012). *Epilepsy surgery in developing countries* (pp. 943–953). https://doi.org/10.1016/B978-0-444-52899-5.00039-3

Collaboration of Industry-Academia-Research-Application Improves the Healthy Development of Medical Imaging Artificial Intelligence Industry in

China. (2019). *Chinese Medical Sciences Journal*, 90. https://doi.org/10.24920/003619

French, J. A., Krauss, G. L., Biton, V., Squillacote, D., Yang, H., Laurenza, A., Kumar, D., & Rogawski, M. A. (2012). Adjunctive perampanel for refractory partial-onset seizures: Randomized phase III study 304. *Neurology, 79*(6), 589–596. https://doi.org/10.1212/WNL.0b013e3182635735

Hannas, W., Chang, H.-M., Chou, D., & Fleeger, B. (2022). *China's Advanced AI Research: Monitoring China's Paths to "General" Artificial Intelligence.* https://doi.org/10.51593/20210064

Jin, B., Li, L., & Rousseau, R. (2004). Long-term influences of interventions in the normal development of science: China and the Cultural Revolution. *Journal of the American Society for Information Science and Technology, 55*(6), 544–550. https://doi.org/10.1002/asi.20010

Jinzhi, Z., & Carrick, J. (2019). The Rise of the Chinese Unicorn: An Exploratory Study of Unicorn Companies in China. *Emerging Markets Finance and Trade*, *55*(15), 3371–3385. https://doi.org/10.1080/1540496X.2019.1610877

Li, Q., Chen, X. Y., He, L., & Zhou, D. (2014). Traditional Chinese medicine for epilepsy. *Cochrane Database of Systematic Reviews*. https://doi.org/10.1002/14651858.CD006454.pub3

Li, Y., Ding, Y., Xiao, W., & Zhu, J.-B. (2021). Investigation on the active ingredient and mechanism of Cannabis sativa L. for treating epilepsy based on network pharmacology. *Biotechnology & Biotechnological Equipment*, *35*(1), 994–1009. https://doi.org/10.1080/13102818.2021.1942208

Lin, C.-H., & Hsieh, C.-L. (2021). Chinese Herbal Medicine for Treating Epilepsy. *Frontiers in Neuroscience*, *15*. https://doi.org/10.3389/fnins.2021.682821

Lin, Y., Hu, S., Hao, X., Duan, L., Wang, W., Zhou, D., Wang, X., Xiao, B., Liu, X., Wang, Y., Zhou, L., Fu, X., Jiang, Y., Zhang, J., Deng, Y., Wang, W., Wu, X., Fang, X., Hong, Z., … Wang, Y. (2021). Epilepsy centers in China : Current status and ways forward. *Epilepsia*, *62*(11), 2640–2650. https://doi.org/10.1111/epi.17058

Men, L. R., Ji, Y. G., & Chen, Z. F. (2019). The state of startups and entrepreneurship in China. In *Strategic Communication for Startups and Entrepreneurs in China* (pp. 11–20). Routledge. https://doi.org/10.4324/9780429274268-2

Minamil, E., Shibata, H., Nunoura, Y., Nomoto, M., & Fukuda, T. (1999). Efficacy of Shitei-To, a Traditional Chinese Medicine Formulation, Against Convulsions in Mice. *The American Journal of Chinese Medicine*, *27*(01), 107–115. https://doi.org/10.1142/S0192415X99000136

Nishida, T., Lee, S. K., Inoue, Y., Saeki, K., Ishikawa, K., & Kaneko, S. (2018). Adjunctive perampanel in partial-onset seizures: Asia-Pacific, randomized phase III study. *Acta Neurologica Scandinavica*, *137*(4), 392–399. https://doi.org/10.1111/ane.12883

Qiu, J. (2016). Research and development of artificial intelligence in China. *National Science Review*, *3*(4), 538–541. https://doi.org/10.1093/nsr/nww076

Qiu, W., Chu, C., Mao, A., & Wu, J. (2018). The Impacts on Health, Society, and Economy of SARS and H7N9 Outbreaks in China: A Case Comparison Study. *Journal of Environmental and Public Health*, *2018*, 1–7. https://doi.org/10.1155/2018/2710185

Roberts, H., Cowls, J., Morley, J., Taddeo, M., Wang, V., & Floridi, L. (2021). The Chinese approach to artificial intelligence: an analysis of policy, ethics, and regulation. *AI & SOCIETY*, *36*(1), 59–77. https://doi.org/10.1007/s00146-020-00992-2

Sander, J. (2008). Gloal campaign against epilepsy: assessment of a demonstration project in rural China. *Bulletin of the World Health Organization*, *86*(12), 964–969. https://doi.org/10.2471/BLT.07.047050

Sander, J. W., & Shorvon, S. D. (1996). Epidemiology of the epilepsies. *Journal of Neurology, Neurosurgery & Psychiatry*, *61*(5), 433–443. https://doi.org/10.1136/jnnp.61.5.433

Thomas, S., & Nair, A. (2011). Confronting the stigma of epilepsy. *Annals of Indian Academy of Neurology*, *14*(3), 158. https://doi.org/10.4103/0972-2327.85873

van der Poest Clement, E. A., Sahin, M., & Peters, J. M. (2018). Vigabatrin for Epileptic Spasms and Tonic Seizures in Tuberous Sclerosis Complex. *Journal of Child Neurology*, *33*(8), 519–524. https://doi.org/10.1177/0883073818768309

Wang, L. (2018). Drug discovery in China: challenges and opportunities. *National Science Review*, *5*(5), 768–773. https://doi.org/10.1093/nsr/nwy085

Wang, Q. (1996). Advances in treatment of epilepsy with traditional Chinese medicine. *Journal of Traditional Chinese Medicine = Chung i Tsa Chih Ying Wen Pan*, *16*(3), 230–237. http://www.ncbi.nlm.nih.gov/pubmed/9389127

Wang, W. Z., Wu, J. Z., Wang, D. S., Dai, X. Y., Yang, B., Wang, T. P., Yuan, C. L., Scott, R. A., Prilipko, L. L., de Boer, H. M., & Sander, J. W. (2003). The prevalence and treatment gap in epilepsy in China: An ILAE/IBE/WHO study. *Neurology*, *60*(9), 1544–1545. https://doi.org/10.1212/01.WNL.0000059867.35547.DE

Wu, Y., Pan, Y., Zhang, Y., Ma, Z., Pang, J., Guo, H., Xu, B., & Yang, Z. (2004). China Scientific and Technical Papers and Citations (CSTPC): History, impact and outlook. *Scientometrics*, *60*(3), 385–397. https://doi.org/10.1023/B:SCIE.0000034381.64865.2b

Xie, Y., Zhang, C., & Lai, Q. (2014). China's rise as a major contributor to science and technology. *Proceedings of the National Academy of Sciences*, *111*(26), 9437–9442. https://doi.org/10.1073/pnas.1407709111

Yamamoto, T., Lim, S. C., Ninomiya, H., Kubota, Y., Shin, W. C., Kim, D. W., Shin, D. J., Hoshida, T., Iida, K., Ochiai, T., Matsunaga, R., Higashiyama, H., Hiramatsu, H., & Kim, J. H. (2020). Efficacy and safety of perampanel monotherapy in patients with focal-onset seizures with newly diagnosed epilepsy or recurrence of epilepsy after a period of remission: The open-label Study 342 (FREEDOM Study). *Epilepsia Open*, *5*(2), 274–284. https://doi.org/10.1002/epi4.12398

Yang, J. (2013). Application of Computer-Aided Drug Design to Traditional Chinese Medicine.

International Journal of Organic Chemistry, *03*(01), 1–16. https://doi.org/10.4236/ijoc.2013.31A001

Yang, R.-R., Wang, W.-Z., Snape, D., Chen, G., Zhang, L., Wu, J.-Z., Baker, G. A., Zheng, X.-Y., & Jacoby, A. (2011). Stigma of people with epilepsy in China: Views of health professionals, teachers, employers, and community leaders. *Epilepsy & Behavior*, *21*(3), 261–266. https://doi.org/10.1016/j.yebeh.2011.04.001

Yang, X. (2019). Accelerated Move for AI Education in China. *ECNU Review of Education*, *2*(3), 347–352. https://doi.org/10.1177/2096531119878590

www.ingramcontent.com/pod-product-compliance
Lightning Source LLC
Chambersburg PA
CBHW050011230526
45465CB00003BB/1372